What you should know about Lung Cancer

Table of Contents

Dedication's Page

This book is dedicated to every patient that may have been diagnosed with lung cancer.

This book Is also dedicated to my beloved father that died from lung cancer.

This book is also dedicated to every medical professional that gives their time to their patients to try and help them through a lung cancer ordeal.

The Basics for Understanding Lung Cancer

Lung cancer is one of the most preventable diseases in the United States.

Lung cancer is also the leading cause of death here in the United States.

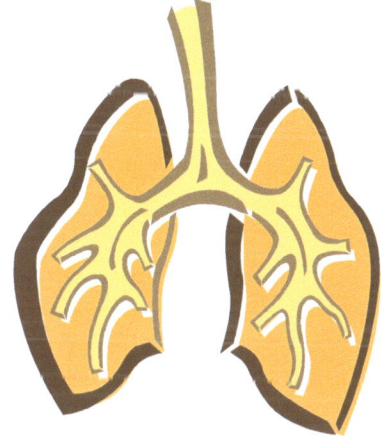

Cigarette smoking leads to four out of five individual cases of people that are diagnosed with lung cancer.

During the 1920's, a large number of males began to smoke cigarettes. Some people began to believe it was due to the large amount of cigarette advertising that was done. Statistics show that after twenty years, there were a huge number of men that was diagnosed with lung cancer.

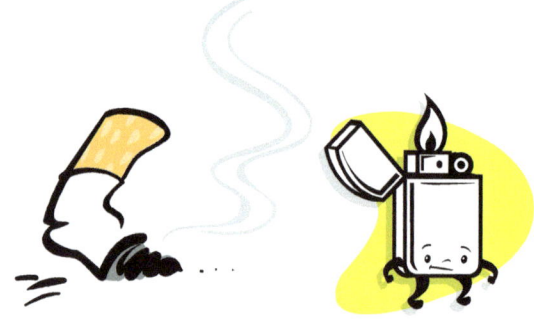

In the 1940's, a huge amount of
women began smoking.
Some people say that it was again due
to the huge amount of advertising
that was performed for the large
cigarette chains.
Twenty years later, there were a large
amount of women that was
diagnosed with lung cancer.

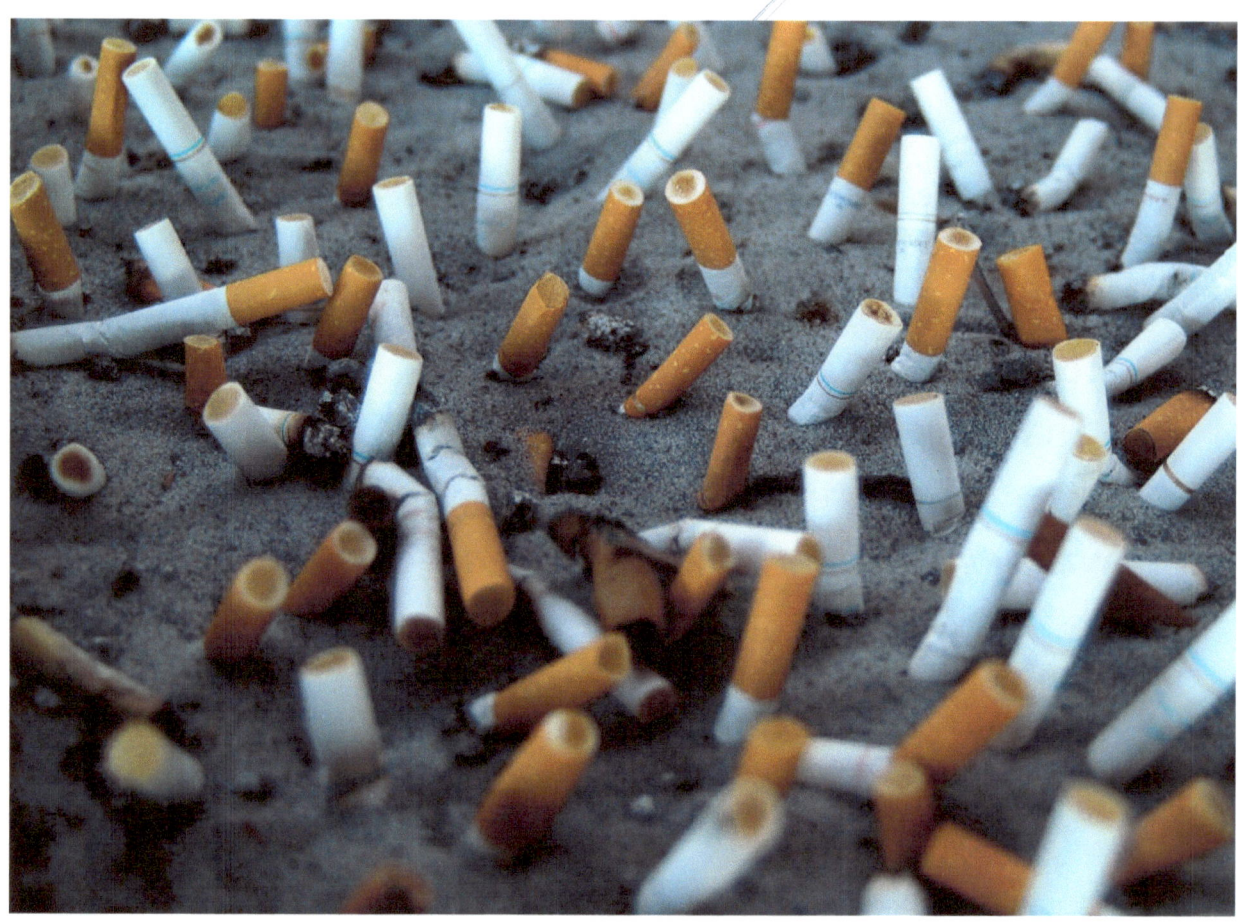

Tumors of the lungs generally always start in the bronchi of the lung. This would be the grayish, pink walls that start the branches of the lungs. The branches are the tubular airways in both of the lungs.

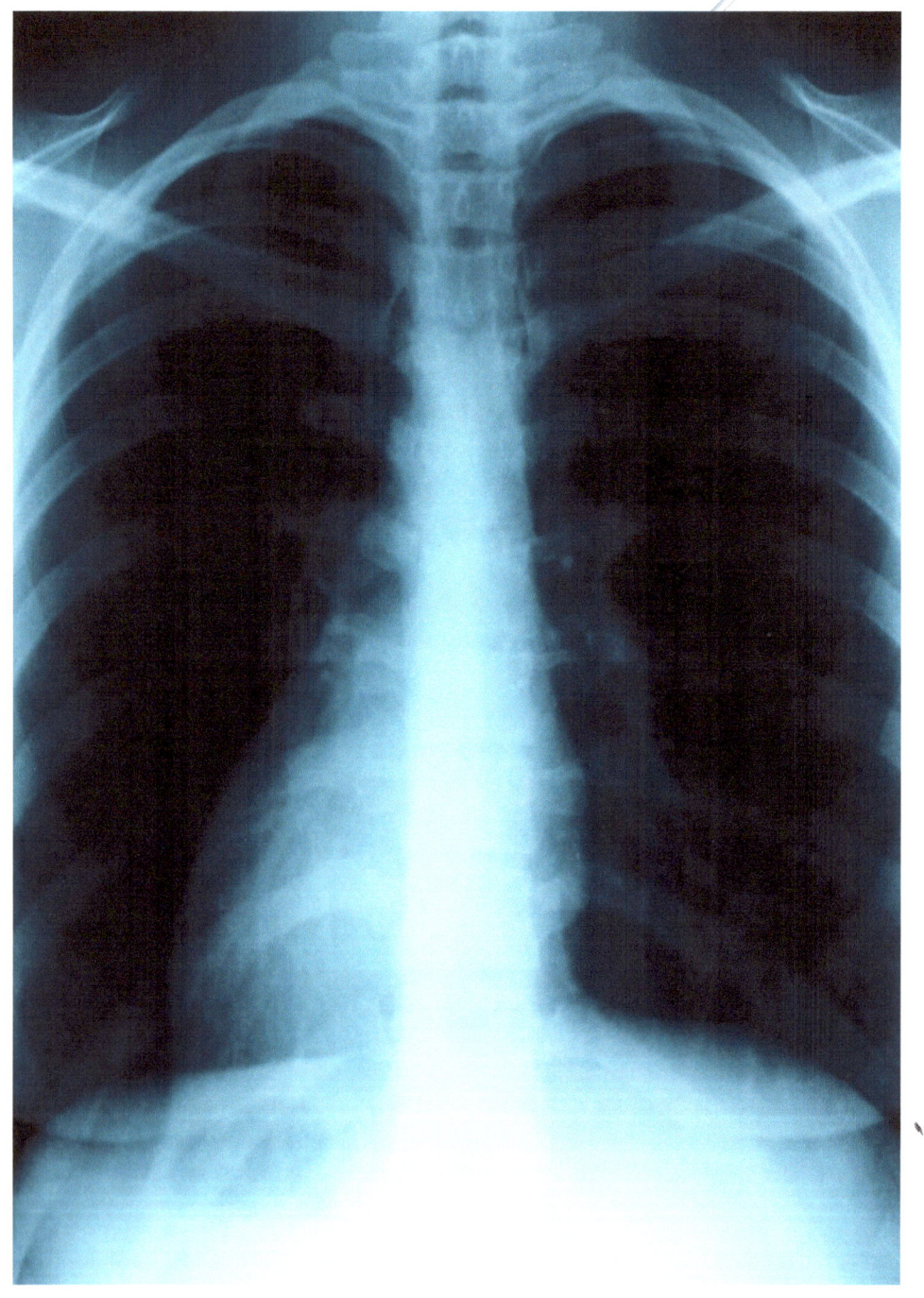

There are basically two types of Lung Cancer:

Small-cell lung cancer and Non-small cell lung cancer

Non-small cell lung cancer types:

- Squamous cell carcinoma generally causes 30 % of the lung cancers and it occurs more commonly in men who are smokers
- It is the easiest to diagnose
- Starts in the cells of the central bronchi tree
- Easiest to cure if found early

Adenocarcinoma

- Most common type of lung cancer
- Generally accounts for about 40 % of all lung cancers diagnosed
- Occurs mainly in people that are currently smoking or have previously smoked in their lifetime
- Statistics say that this type of cancer generally occurs in younger adults and more commonly in woman

Large-cell carcinoma

- Large-cell carcinoma tends to originate along the outer edges of a person's lungs
- This type of lung cancer generally only accounts for 10%-15% of all diagnosed patients
- This type of cancer spreads to distant sites and a person's lymph nodes

Small-cell Lung Cancer

- This type of lung cancer is the most aggressive form
- It does not typically allow long term survival
- In over 75% of all patients that are diagnosed, this type of lung cancer generally metastasizes to the brain, liver and their bones
- This is the second leading cancer in both of the sexes, both male and females
- It kills 160,000 people per year

What causes Lung Cancer?

Smoking causes about 85% of all
lung cancer.
A person's genetics is also a
contributing factor.
The fact that a person has a
family history of cancer is almost
predisposition that they could
inherit cancer.

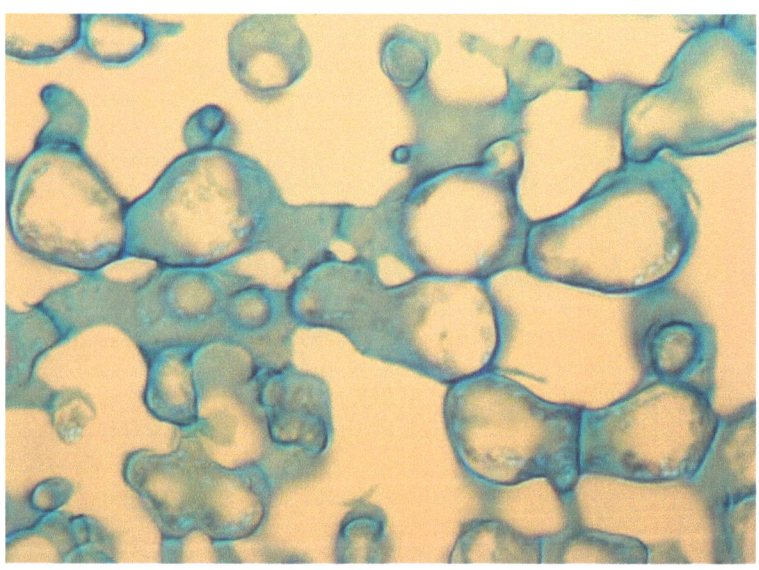

Any person that smokes a pack of cigarettes per day is 20 times more likely to obtain lung cancer in their lifetime than a non-smoker.

A person that smokes two packs per day, their risk triples for obtaining lung cancer in their lifetime than that of a non-smoker.

If a person quits smoking, their risks decrease, but smokers are always more susceptible than non-smokers.

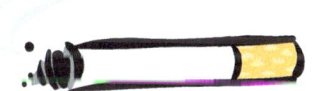

Lung cancer can also be caused
by second-hand smoke.
Non-smokers who live or work
with smokers are at a higher risk
of obtaining lung cancer that
those that are in a smoke-free
environment.

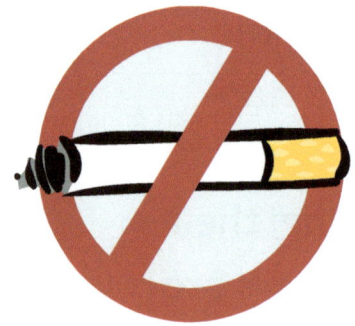

Those living in a home environment with a person that may smoke have over a 30% chance of obtaining lung cancer in their lifetime.
Second-hand smoke contributed to over 3,000 deaths just last year.

Cancer-causing substances can also cause lung cancer. Asbestos attributes to about a 90 fold chance of obtaining lung cancer. People who work around uranium dust or radioactive gas radon can also get lung cancer. People that work around these cancer-causing substances have a huge chance of obtaining this deadly disease than a person that does not work in these types of environment.

If a person has been exposed to an infection or some sort of disease that has caused scarring on their lungs, they could also be more susceptible to obtain lung cancer that someone else.

An example could be tuberculosis or scleroderma.

A tumor can grow in the scarred portions of the lungs caused by the disease or the infection.

People who eat large amounts of fatty foods or who have high cholesterol could obtain this disease as well over time.

Lung Cancer Symptoms

In the early stages of lung cancer, some people experience no symptoms at all.

However, over time, they could experience these symptoms:

- Difficult swallowing
- Weakness or pain In their hands, arms, or shoulders
- Raspy breathing with bloody mucus
- Recurrent respiratory infections like pneumonia or bronchitis
- Shortness of breath or some coughing
- Hoarseness

Lung Cancer Diagnoses

Lung Cancer Diagnoses can be made by:

- Facial edema
- Expanded veins in the head, neck and check regions of the body
- Abnormal sounds in the person's lungs
- Rounding of the person's fingernails
- A mass in the person's abdomen
- Weak breathing

Lung Cancer Testing Procedures

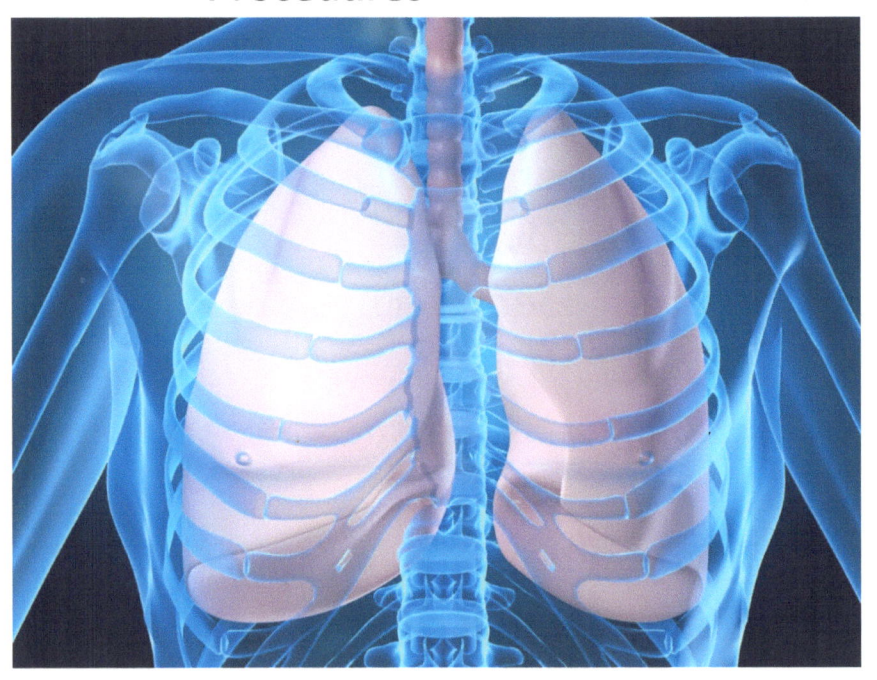

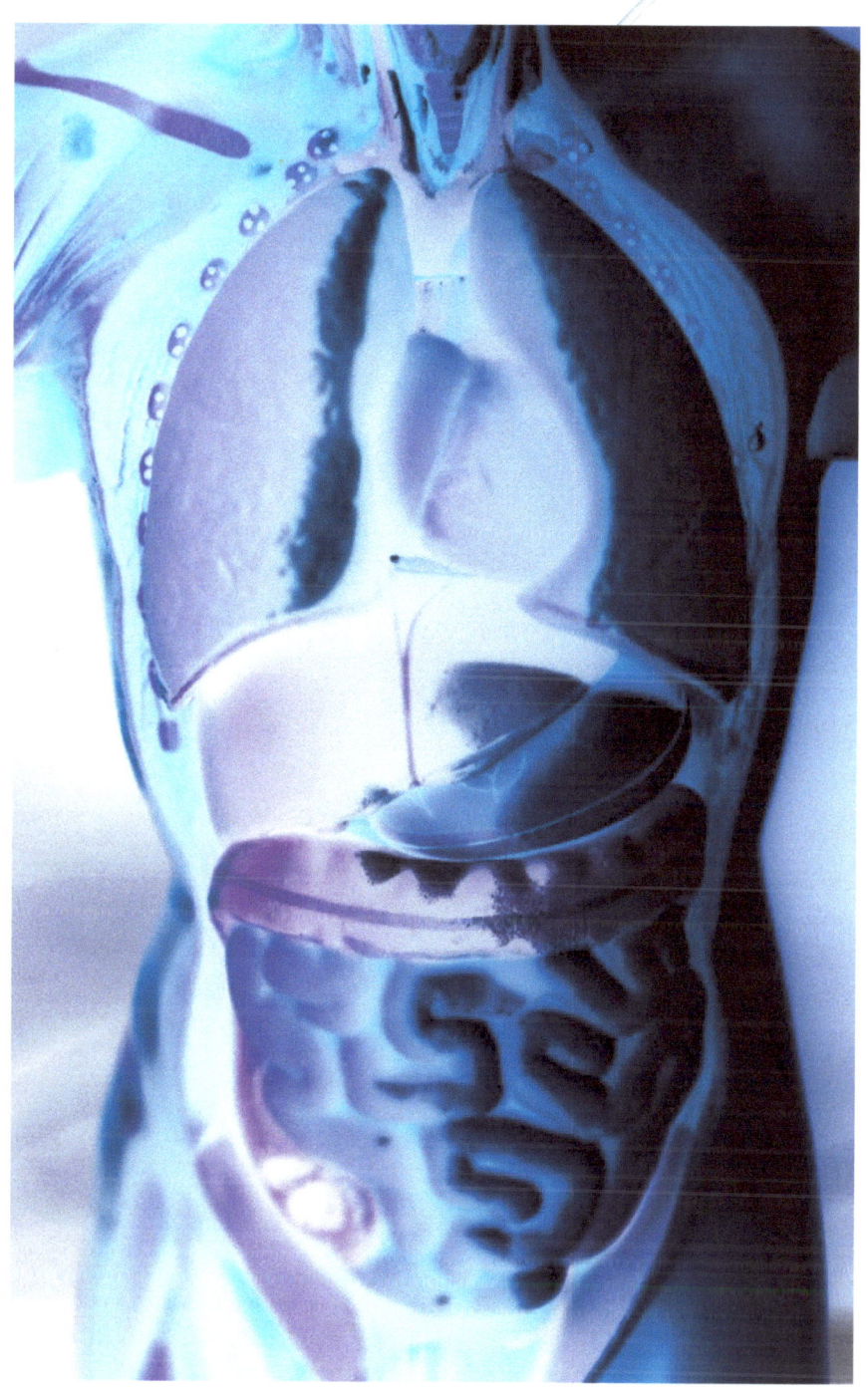

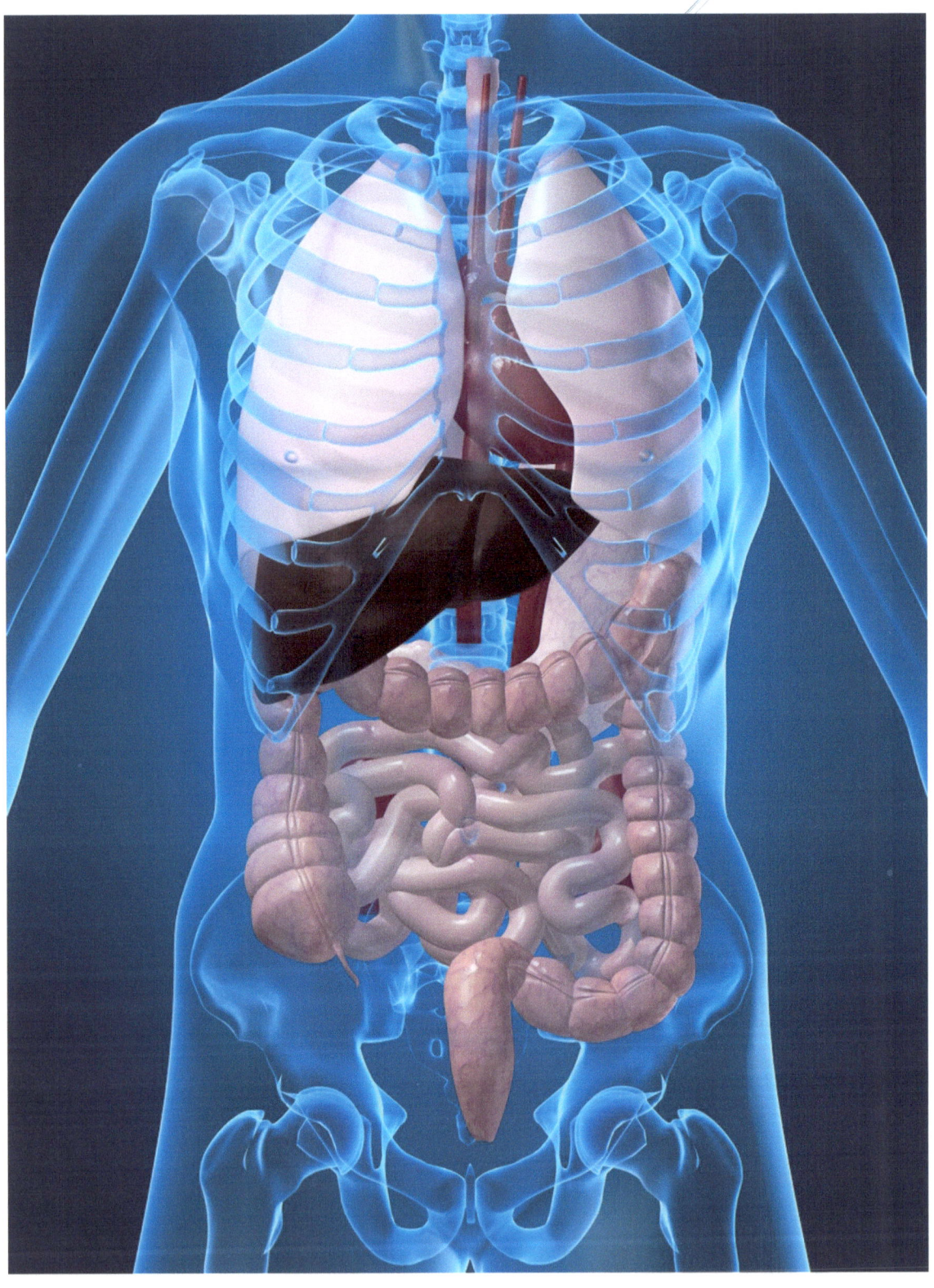

Some tests could be as follows:
- A lung biopsy
- Lung sputum cytology
- A lung pet scan
- Bone scans
- A Cat Scan of the Brain to diagnose Lung Cancer

Conclusions

By reading this material and becoming familiar with the statistics, a person could decrease their risks for obtaining lung cancer and have a happy and much healthier life.

What You Should Know about Lung Cancer is a self-help guide to helping an individual understand about their disease and its statistics? This book also gives some insight into the types of lung cancer and how the disease can spread to other areas of the body. The book also gives some insight into how your physician may diagnose lung cancer and some of the testing procedures that they may perform.

Misty Lynn Wesley has a diversified career portfolio in the medical, legal, fashion and insurance industries. She is an avid blogger for Examiner.com and she also writes for CBS Local out of St. Paul, Minnesota and Believe.com sometimes. She has since been given another promotion to AXS as well. She has written four books with Publish America and she has written several books on Amazon. She and her chosen producers have also made

several audio books which can be found on
Amazon, Barnes and Noble and I tunes.
God bless and enjoy!